The Experiment

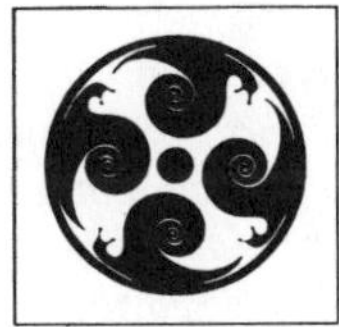

by Renée Brand

C. G. Jung Institute of
San Francisco

Published by the C. G. Jung Institute of San Francisco, Inc.
2040 Gough Street, San Francisco, California 94109

Grateful acknowledgment for permission to reprint copyrighted material is made to Princeton University Press for quotations from *The Collected Works of C. G. Jung,* edited by G. Adler, M. Fordham, and H. Read; translated by R. F. C. Hull; Bollingen Series XX, vol. 16; copyright © 1954

Abbreviation of Principal Reference

CW = *The Collected Works of C. G. Jung.* Edited by Gerhard Adler, Michael Fordham, and Herbert Read; William McGuire, Executive Editor; translated by R. F. C. Hull; New York and Princeton (Bollingen Series XX) and London, 1953-1978. 20 vols. References are to paragraph numbers.

Design and mechanicals by Robert Sibley.
Type set in Garamond 3 by Abracadabra, San Francisco.
Printed and bound by Fremont Litho, Fremont, California.

Printed in the United States of America
ISBN 0-932630-02-2

FOREWORD

For most analysands, transference as experience is at its core an ineffable mystery. This is equally true of the analyst's experience of countertransference when the analyst is touched by the analytic relationship at the frontier of his or her own unfolding in the depths of human experience. The analytic relationship is ". . . a human encounter where love plays the decisive part."[1] As such, it is touched by ". . . the fatal touch of incest and its 'perverse' fascination."[2] Jung says, "Incest symbolizes union with one's own being, it means individuation or becoming a self, and, because this is so vitally important, it exerts an unholy fascination—not, perhaps, as a crude reality, but certainly as a psychic process controlled by the unconscious . . ."[3]

The word *transference* usually connotes a familiar clinical situation which Jung described as follows:

> The conventional meeting [of analyst with analysand] is followed by an unconscious "familiarization" of [the analyst by the analysand], brought about by the projection of archaic, infantile fantasies which were originally vested in members of the patient's own family and which, because of their positive or negative fascination, attach him to parents, brothers, and sisters. The transference of these fantasies to the doctor draws him into the atmosphere of family intimacy, and although this is the last thing he wants, it nevertheless provides a work-

---

[1] CW 16, Par. 419.

[2] Ibid.

[3] Ibid.

> able *prima materia.* Once the transference has appeared, the doctor must accept it as part of the treatment and try to understand it, otherwise it will be just another piece of neurotic stupidity. The transference itself is a perfectly natural phenomenon which does not by any means happen only in the consulting room—it can be seen everywhere and may lead to all sorts of nonsense, like all unrecognized projections. Medical treatment of the transference gives the patient a priceless opportunity to withdraw his projections, to make good his losses, and to integrate his personality.[4]

The limitation of this conception of the transference is that it is too linear, too rationally conceived, implying a series of steps to be taken which, of course, every experienced therapist should understand, follow, and convey to the patient in a series of properly timed, rational interpretations. In this conception, what the analyst must accept and analyze is the transference neurosis—"another piece of neurotic stupidity." Of course, we all strive to analyze our transference neuroses away. However, as the neurotic projections of personal images are withdrawn and integrated, we are still left with a "transference," an infusion of the analytic relationship with the Self and what Michael Fordham has called its deintegrates. That is, the analytic relationship is guided by the principle of wholeness, and the analyst continues to "carry" for or "represent" for the analysand those aspects of the Self with which the patient needs to develop a relation until they can be integrated into a realized selfhood. Since both the analysand and the analyst participate in the Self and share an encounter with the archetypes of the collective unconscious, the image of an incestuous union is an apt one, vitalized by feelings of love which are not to be concretized.

Renée Brand is a Jungian analyst and a creative writer. In *The Experiment,* she uses her literary imagination to convey an experience of transference as an experiment, consciously entered into, which becomes an unbidden and irrevocable commitment to a process infinitely larger than the narrator. She provides a picture of transference as an inner containment of this process, "The Room," a place where significant things happen even when they are imaginary. She reveals a peculiar sensitivity to the nature of symbolism, which combines reality and fantasy in a way that does justice to both.

Both by education and temperament, Dr. Brand is well fitted to

---

[4]Ibid, par. 420.

understand and express the use of symbolism in Jungian thought and psychoanalysis. As a very young woman in Germany, she was thrust by marriage to a substantially older, prominent industrialist into a highly cultivated world of artists, writers, architects of the Weimar Republic. She was mistress of a great house designed by their friend Walter Gropius and came under the influence of her husband's friends from an older generation. It was a time of a rising generation of writers determined to throw over the old order, such as Myrinck, Hesse, Mann, and of daring experimenters represented at the Bauhaus, where beside the new architecture of Gropius and his students, the painters Kandinsky and Klee were experimenting with visual symbolism that was destined to inform a whole new direction in painting. Renée Brand was responsive to the indirect, symbolic style of Kafka and other writers who wrote not only novels, but *feuilletons* which fired imagination and freed the mind from prejudice.

This period of German creativity was swept away by the Nazi movement, and many whose art was just beginning to be formed had to go into exile. Renée Brand made of this tragic period a saving transition. She fled Germany for France at the last possible moment, the Nazis at her heels. Eventually, she was able to obtain residency in Switzerland and settled in Basel. In Basel she studied at the University in a more or less casual way and wrote a novel entitled *Niemandsland* (No-Man's Land),[5] inspired by her period of waiting for resident status in Switzerland. The novel was conceived and written in the symbolic style I have mentioned and is about a group of Germans who have been expelled from Germany but have not yet acquired asylum in a neighboring country such as Holland or Switzerland. The novel describes their life in the wretched piece of country where they had to camp for many weeks until they could be accepted into the new country. The various members of the group have different reactions, but in one way or another, they each affirm an old cultural value that may be renewed in their future home.

As she continued her studies at the University of Basel over a period of years, she was eventually encouraged by her professors, Walter Muschg and Friedrich Ranke, to focus upon completing a Ph.D. degree in literature and philosophy. Her dissertation was entitled *Zur Interpretation des "Ackermann aus Böhmen"* and was published in 1942

[5]Zurich: Oprecht, 1940.

by Benno Schwabe and Company of Basel. In the meantime, her novel enjoyed considerable success in German and was translated into English under the title *Short Days Ago,*[6] and she was invited to come to the United States. She arrived in New York on a wave of literary acclaim. Here began another period of painful transition in which she could not find work in keeping with her background and quickly learned that she was unable to write in English at a literary level. It was in these first years in the United States that she discovered Jungian psychology, and the forces which led to her becoming an analyst were set in motion.

The theme of transition, so deeply experienced in her life and so sensitively treated in her novel, forms the basis of her understanding of transference as an experience of disorientation and possible suffering through which old values come into new life. Growing out of this history, *The Experiment* is doubly real and powerfully evocative of the experience of transference in analysis and conveys its essential meaning without interpretation because, like transference itself, it may mean something different to each reader.

There remains, however, one element which is constant in such experience: the love the analysand and the analyst feel for one another is not personally concretized, and this is the necessary condition from which may arise in the analysand a new capacity to love which had never before been possible. With the experience of this love comes a new conviction that we do not live from ego consciousness alone but by a significant union of ego with the Self.

> Now is the stone shaped, the elixir of life prepared, the love-child or the child of love, the new birth completed, and the work made whole and perfect. Farewell! Fall, hell, curse, death, dragon, beast, and serpent! Good night! Mortality, fear, sorrow, and misery! For now redemption, salvation, and recovery of everything that was lost will come again to pass within and without, for now you have the great secret and mystery of the whole world; you have the Pearl of Love; you have the unchangeable eternal essence of Divine Joy from which all healing virtue and all multiplying power come, from which there actively proceeds the active power of the Holy Ghost. You have the seed of the woman who has trampled on the head of the serpent. You have the seed of the virgin and the blood of the virgin in one essence and quality.[7]

---

[6] New York: Farrar, 1941.

[7] From a letter by John Pordage to his *sorror mystica* Jane Leade, published in 1698, and quoted by Jung in CW 16, par. 516.

At this point, a resolution of the transference to the analyst is made possible, and a separation from the analytic process is made. This is accomplished not without a deep sense of loss at parting, but with a reassurance that the experience of the analytic relationship has become a permanent acquisition of the capacity to live both humanly and symbolically in accordance with that experience.

In *The Experiment,* Dr. Brand brings this alive with particular poignancy in the narrator's death experience, which would appear to flow directly from the incestuous intensity of the transference union. "[O]ne cannot rid oneself of the impression that death is a sort of tacit punishment for the sin of incest, for 'the wages of sin is death.' That would explain the soul's 'great distress' . . . . "[8] Dr. Brand's development of this theme is particularly touching and true to life experience; one senses that the transference is not completely "resolved," that subtle threads of regressive longing remain amid the conscious suffering of sacrifice of the relationship and the embracing of life.

Dr. Brand brought *The Experiment* together from two fragments of larger works-in-progress for oral presentation. Changes from second to third person have been made in Chapter III for greater clarity and consistency as a written presentation, and changes in punctuation and minor phrasings have been made throughout to conform with standard English usage.

In recent years, Renée Brand has been retired from the practice of Jungian analysis, though she has been the inspiratrice for and, until recently, the Advisory Editor of the "Neumann Project," the translation of Erich Neumann's previously untranslated papers being published by Princeton University Press under the sponsorship of the C. G. Jung Institute of San Francisco.[9] Through Dr. Joseph L. Henderson, who has collaborated in the writing of this foreword, *The Experiment* came to light as uniquely expressive of Dr. Brand and her relation to analytical psychology. With this publication, the C. G. Jung Institute of San Francisco is privileged to honor Renée Brand as she ends her long career, in recognition of her many years of service to the Institute and its programs.

Gareth S. Hill
Berkeley, California
October, 1980

---

[8] CW 16, par. 468.

[9] The first volume has appeared as *Creative Man; Five Essays,* Bollingen Series LXI: 2. Princeton, N.J.: Princeton University Press, 1979.

The Experiment

I.

There was a moment when I thought I could choose whether or not to get into The Experiment. I was convinced it was my decision, and I can remember how I stood there wondering whether I should or shouldn't and thinking that it would be a daring thing indeed to expose myself to the disease in order to find out more definitely about the serum. Of course, I had complete faith in The Experiment and also in the skill of the scientist with whom it would be carried out. And even at that time I was obsessed with The Experiment; it seemed the only worthwhile thing in life. So it would have been very difficult not to get involved more deeply.

I believed that it was sheer scientific interest that compelled me, and the desire to make a contribution to this cause—not just *a* contribution, but the one contribution I could make and therefore had to make. So, my partner and I signed the pact. And like all such pacts, from time immemorial, this one too was signed with blood. One can easily see that the Devil got into it right then and there: two people sitting down one sober summer morning in a modern big city to get together on a scientific experiment, both stating what their roles in the work would have to be, and one of them—myself—signing the agreement with blood. That isn't a very up-to-date way of doing things; it has a medieval flavor. It should have made me wary of the consequences. If the Devil gets into such pacts, one might lose one's soul. The actual time-honored procedure for such signatures has been for the two partners to open their veins and dip their pens into them, the way boys do at the scouting age. But in cases where it is a question of the Devil Himself, there is only one who signs with the precious liquid. However, it isn't immediately possible to know that one might be dealing with forces such as the Devil or God. We know very little, and our scientific training has made us very skeptical.

Of course, there was no Devil around that particular morning. There were two perfectly inconspicuous scientists, a man and a woman, and the business about signing a pact with blood did not enter into it at all. We did not sign any agreements in reality, nor open any veins. That would have been a perfectly monstrous idea; it never occurred to us. But I volunteered to formulate something very close to a pact. I said I would give myself to The Experiment. I would simply give myself up to it. At the same time I would try to observe scientifically the happenings within my own living organism, so as to make the specific contribution I felt called upon to make to the science. I also said I would make these observations fully known to my partner, so that we could use them as seemed necessary and right. For this purpose, I committed myself to keep records of my condition and to make these records available to him without editing or censorship. My capacity to formulate in writing what I feel brought with it this obligation.

I haven't made clear enough the point about signing this pact with my own blood nor, perhaps, the nature of the pact. It was simply that I would make myself available to be experimented on with the help and under the supervision of my partner, the other scientist, and that I would keep these records in which should be expressed the truth, the whole truth, and nothing but the truth about the conditions I would observe while under the effect of The Experiment.

Immediately after I had formulated my role in the work and had put it in writing, something odd happened. (Up to that moment I thought I was free; I could make this agreement or not make it, or figure out a different agreement altogether, or step out of the whole thing. My partner had not made any conditions except the usual ones about which I shall speak later.) It was with my free will and with my eyes open that my own hand had written the agreement, the pact, and I took it to him to decide together whether this was how things were going to be. I found that something had taken place which made it impossible to change anything about it. I could not step out of the thing anymore. I could not change the set-up nor my obligations which were, after all, self-imposed. I found the agreement had become effective the moment it was written down, and it became inalterable the moment he laid eyes on it. I squirmed in my chair. I choked with words of regret and retreat which I could not utter. I was utterly convinced I had made a most serious mistake, yet there was nothing I could do. The matter was settled.

That kind of a situation comes up only when a pact is signed with one's own blood, and when somehow, mysteriously, the Devil has had a hand in it. And God too. For the Devil stands on Low, and God stands on High. And High stands on Low. This is one of the scientific facts one has to deal with in connection with The Experiment.

* * * *

When I came back the following day, my partner showed me The Room. We had to take the elevator down to the basement of the building and then walk along a narrow corridor which was only faintly lit.

This is a big modern office building, and I was surprised to find that this long corridor had but one door at the far end, the door leading to The Room. My partner, U., as I will call him for short, assured me that I would be completely undisturbed, The Room being reserved for our Experiment. Nobody had access to it, and there was no telephone or other connection with the rest of the building. I would be on my own, the way I had to be.

He reminded me that he was within easy reach in his office on the top floor. If anything untoward happened in The Room, it would take but a few minutes to get to him for aid. I smiled. What could happen? I had experimented before, I was not unacquainted with the procedure nor the events I had to expect. Indeed, I prided myself on being well initiated through my previous work. He guessed my thoughts and replied that even he did not anticipate in the least what was going to turn up in our Experiment, in spite of the fact that he had supervised work of this kind for many years. There is no way of knowing, and I should leave myself open to all eventualities.

He also warned me that I might find The Experiment painful. I was prepared to suffer the necessary pain. Everything in life has its price, and I am not hesitant to pay. The experiences in The Room will be more painful in my case, since I am going to operate through my capacity for feeling, whereas most of the other scientists work more intellectually.

U. seemed to be very interested in my promise to keep records of everything. Nobody had been able to do that so far. With great warmth he assured me of his fullest cooperation in every respect and without any reservations.

His personal warmth and interest affected me strongly. I felt again, as I had upon our first meeting, that he was the right man for this undertaking. I had been very fortunate in coming to him. We shook hands like old friends, and it was almost impossible for me to believe that we had just met. U. gave me to understand that there was a more direct connection between The Room in the basement and his office on the top floor. I would not have to rely on the elevator which does not always function. There was a spiral staircase available from within which led directly into his own rooms, but it might be difficult to find, and it would also take some effort to climb up all those stairs. However, it was a good thing to know about.

I had kept the elated mood I had had the day before, and the new assurance of U.'s participation in The Experiment to the full extent of his capacity made me feel I did not need any further preparations but could go right ahead.

We had talked all this time standing in front of the closed door, as, of course, U. could not accompany me into The Room. He then took his leave, congratulating me upon my readiness to go to work immediately and repeating once more that I should not let myself get too troubled by anything that might occur. I watched him walk back through the corridor, and I felt a most pleasant sensation at the easy gracefulness of his slender figure. His poise and carriage accentuated the feeling of harmony his appearance gave me, and I had to control myself not to call out to him to turn around once more for another look at his sensitive face, which had already become dear to me.

But he had disappeared around the corner while I was still debating in my mind whether it was the right thing to do. So I turned back to the closed door and waited silently for a few minutes.

I knew I could not just go ahead and open it. It had a lock similar to the complicated locks we put on a safe door. You have to know the combination of letters and figures and turn it accordingly. It was a question of hitting the right idea. As I stood there trying to collect myself, my thoughts wandered in spite of my effort to keep them together. I felt a strange warmth enveloping me, and I heard faint music whose source I could not immediately locate. Then I was aware that it was coming from within The Room. The theme seemed familiar, and as I listened more carefully, I recognized the first movement of Beethoven's *Appassionata.* Miraculously, the combination for the lock presented itself at that moment, and I opened the door.

* * * *

At first it was impossible to see anything in the dim light of The Room, and I had to wait till my eyes were more accustomed to the semi-darkness. I pulled the door shut and leaned against it, waiting. The music seemed to come from another room which might be connected. It was the most beautiful performance of the sonata I had ever heard. Not only was it played with fire and passion, but there was a clarity of interpretation which made the piece transparent in its structure and brought an element of sublime order and purposefulness to the heightened feeling it released.

I advanced a few steps into The Room and became aware that the light was no longer dim. The Room was a perfect square, and it seemed of great height—in fact, I could not see the ceiling at all; it seemed to go off into space. I realized that that must be an erroneous idea on my part—probably a lack of perception—since this was the basement on which rested the whole building; there must be a ceiling to The Room. There were soft draperies along the walls, or what I guessed must be the walls, for the walls were not visible either. The colors were harmoniously blended and of the most exquisite shades of blue and red, purple and violet, with green and yellow tinges. The silky materials moved faintly as if a light breeze were caught in them, but that might have been the effect of the music. The Room seemed completely empty, except for a very comfortable wing chair in one corner and next to it a small end table with a pad of writing paper and a pen. I went and sat down, closing my eyes and letting myself be carried away by the music whose source was still hidden.

After a few minutes, I felt that the playing sounded closer, and as I opened my eyes again, I saw that in the very center of The Room there was a sunken space, a perfect circle, and while I looked at it, wondering whether it would be possible to get down deeper, into a lower basement perhaps, the circular emptiness was filled; the sunken center was rising to the level at which I sat. It had the effect of a theater trapdoor used to make the actors disappear or appear seemingly out of nowhere.

In the center of the circle sat U. at the piano. It was his playing I had heard. He seemed to be oblivious of my presence and swayed lightly back and forth on his seat, absorbed in the music he was producing.

I was more than pleased to see him and deeply moved by his exquisite performance of this piece I knew so well and loved so dearly. He paused for a moment after the breath-taking crescendos of the first movement, and I wanted to express my appreciation. I rose and walked toward the center where he sat, but as I approached him, I realized that the instrument and he were walled off by a glass enclosure which did not seem to have any opening.

That was impossible. How could he have gotten in unless there were some opening? I called to him, but either he was too absorbed or my voice could not rise above the music—he had started playing the second movement by then; at any rate, he did not hear me. I felt rather frustrated, but I was too grateful for his presence and the unexpected deep pleasure of listening to his playing to allow this feeling of frustration to last.

I went back to my chair and gave myself up to the music, looking at the man as he sat there, swaying in the rhythm of the piece, his eyes unseeing. The spirituality of his face filled me with admiration. I thought he had a beautiful head. He must have known of my presence, but he chose not to give any sign of his awareness; maybe I was to understand that we should not talk.

I kept my eyes on his face, and the more I looked at him, the happier I felt about him. With a sudden shock I realized that the feeling I had was one of love. I tried to convince myself that it could not be so. I did not wish to love this man. It would be the most ridiculous and impractical thing that could possibly happen. It might happen to a beginner, but I had enough previous experience to be able to avoid such time-consuming mistakes as that one. Besides, I did not feel the slightest inclination to fall in love. I had adjusted myself to the life of a professional woman who has established the habit of living alone. I was not interested in love anymore. I was way beyond that stage in life. It would be an unnecessary and painful detour which could not bring any new information, and it might distract my attention from The Experiment. It was also a most impractical thing. U. was married and happy in his marriage. Our relationship was strictly limited to the work we were to do together. I felt quite embarrassed at the thought that this idea had even occurred to me, especially since I would have to put it into the records, which meant that he would know about it.

Well, I could put it in the context of thoughts around it, showing that I understood it would lead nowhere and should not be allowed to happen. I felt some relief at this solution.

My thoughts must have taken me away from the music because I only then became aware that the playing had stopped, and as I looked toward the center I realized that U. had left. The center had dropped down again, and there was the same empty circular space I had noticed when I first came in.

I thought I must have spent a long time in The Room and that it might be as well to leave. I must admit that I was also anxious to get to U. in spite of the discomfort I felt at the thought of having to report to him the occurrence of love. My heart was beating as I knocked at his door, and I reprimanded myself for that. But when he opened the door and asked me in, I felt more relaxed and at ease again.

I thanked him for coming to The Room, in spite of the rules and regulations which demanded that I go there alone, and wondered how he had gotten in. Since I had not been able to discover a second door, yet found him inside, he must have gotten in before me and by some other entrance.

He told me that he had not been in The Room at all. There was no second entrance. He could not get in even if he wished to. The Room was strictly reserved for me; nobody else was able to get in. It must have been another man, possibly looking much like him but belonging to The Room. Only the people belonging to The Room could be found in it.

I argued this point at length. I knew that I would meet in The Room the people who belong there. But I also knew I had seen him, and no error was possible. I could not get him to admit that he indeed had gotten in, but I saw a smile in his eyes, and I thought he might not wish to discuss it openly. I decided I must not press the point any further and just be grateful to him for coming. So I agreed to speak of the "Man in The Room" as if that had been someone else who resembled U.

We discussed the glass enclosure which had made it impossible for me to communicate with the man at the piano. He thought it was a shame that I had been unable to get through to the man, and he promised me that he would help me find a way. This was the very first thing U. wanted to do. He would remove the obstacle, so that the man and I could get together. I had expected criticism as I felt responsible for the things happening in The Room. But he assured me I need not fear any criticism on his part. He was well aware that I had not put the glass there. It was there. It would have to be taken away. He would give me a hand in this since it would be too difficult for me to get it out of the way alone.

I reminded myself that the man I was supposed to get together with was actually U. himself, not just a man, and my heart started acting up again. But I did not say anything about it, accepting it the way he wanted me to, agreeing it was not himself but some man who looked like him.

At this point I found the courage to tell him that a feeling very much like love had occurred as I sat listening to the music. I added that I well knew it could not really be love and that I had everything under control.

He smiled his heart-warming smile again and looked at me silently for a few minutes. I felt myself melting away under his smile and wondered how well I would be able to exert the necessary control. "Is it up to you?" he asked.

This was a strange question. Of course it was up to me.

"How can one 'control' a feeling? Have you made it? Or did it happen to you? Did you put the glass enclosure around the man who played? Or did you find it there?"

"I thought I am responsible."

"You are responsible for finding what is there and looking at what is there."

There was silence. I was acutely aware of my ineffectual fencing. I had mentioned before that I signed a pact and that it was signed with my blood. It seemed I did not have any choice in the matter. Yet the very thought of allowing myself to love this man made me squirm. This was where the Devil came in, I thought. This was an aspect of the agreement I had not bargained for.

"You are a woman. Life reveals itself to you through your feeling. You have to accept your feeling, as I accept it. You must not be afraid of The Experiment. Do not fear."

His voice was gentle and strong. His words touched me at the core. I looked up and looked at the man who had this voice and these words. I looked straight into his eyes, and he looked back at me. There was a stream of fire, and the moment became Eternity.

"You do not have to fight against it," he said ever so gently.

I tore my eyes away from him and looked down at my hands which were twisted in my lap. His regard followed me and rested on my hands. They opened as the petals of a flower under the rays of the sun and lay down peacefully. I saw they were a woman's hands. I felt my body from the tingling roots of my hair to the tips of my toes which were allowed to rest firmly on the floor. It was a woman's body, and it heaved a sigh.

"Do not fear," he said, "all will be well."

I could not answer; the words choked me. My voice was gone.

There was a stirring in the depth of my womb. I received his seed into me in immaculate conception.

When I was able to look at him again, I saw U. sitting across from me, patiently waiting. His brow was touched with light, and his eyes were illuminated.

"We have to be humble," he said, "The Experiment is under way. All will be well, *Deo Concedente.*"

"Deo Concedente," I answered, almost inaudibly. And to myself I added: *"Amor Fati."*

"You may want to leave now to start the records. The records will be helpful so that we can have the testimony of the word, and language is given you for that purpose."

He gave me his hand, and I left.

* * * *

As I got out on the street and into the clear light of this summer afternoon, I felt dizzy and confused. The busy noise of the city drowned out his words, and my thoughts became blurred. I crossed the street and went into a coffee-shop.

The people at the counter, the people at the tables, eating, chatting, the clamor of traffic outside: I felt I had no part in it all—it was spooky—but I did not know if I were the ghost or they. I tried to talk sense to myself. This, I told myself, is nothing but an experiment. Life as I see it around me is real. The other: What kind of thing is that? Are there words for it? What kind of words?

I had thought: the immaculate conception. And what does that mean? Scientifically speaking, there is no such thing. Surely, I like this man, U. But that is no reason to put it in such fantastic, irrational terms. Look at this girl; she is eating a doughnut with her coffee and talking to her friend eagerly, with her mouth full. What are they talking about?

"I am not sure if he is thinking of marriage. He hasn't said anything. I can't figure him out. I am not going to let myself get involved any more deeply. I am simply not going to. I have to know where I'm at. That's all there is to it."

She is right. She is not going to let herself get involved. She has to know where "she's at." That's plain common sense. Let's use a little common sense, too. Let's keep each thing in its place. The Experiment has its place and so has life. Let's not get it mixed up, for heaven's sake.

I got into my car to drive home. Home right then was a place in the country which I had rented for the time I was going to give to The Experiment so that I would be able to concentrate without external disturbance.

As I drove along, the world outside receded again. I looked at my hands at the wheel, and I had the same strange new feeling about them: a woman's hands.

I brushed against the shrubbery, walking through the garden and up to the house and feeling the touch of cool leaves at my fingers. The feeling persisted. I took the food out of the refrigerator and started to prepare supper. The feeling remained. It was as if everything I touched responded to my hands with almost a caress. Or was it that a new tenderness had come into my hands?

I smelled the sourdough bread, and it smelt like fresh earth. Before sitting down to eat, I went outside again to pick some flowers. The garden, too, smelt of fresh earth. Hummingbirds were alighting in the fruit trees, and watching them with fascination, I forgot that I had the food on the table waiting for me. I sat down on the porch, looking at the mountain across the valley. It was clearly outlined against the paling sky and luminous from the sun setting behind it. Fear gripped me. I was helpless against it. A chill went through me. It might have been the cool evening air, but then I heard his voice. U. said: Do not fear. And another voice, one I had never heard, said: Do not kill the seed.

After dinner I sat down by the fire with a book. The old book felt strange in my new hands. I had thumbed through it many times, opening it here and there at random. Following the old habit, I let it fall open and looked at the page.

Hast thou commanded the morning since thy days began, And caused the dayspring to know its place[?]

[Is it up to you?]

Hast thou entered into the springs of the sea?
Or hast thou walked in the recesses of the deep?

[Is it up to you?]

Has thou comprehended the breadth of the earth?
—Declare if thou knowest it all—
Where is the way to the dwelling of light,
And as for darkness, where is the place thereof;
That thou shouldest take it to the bound thereof,
And that thou shouldest discern the paths to the house thereof?

[Is it up to you?]

Canst thou bind the clusters of the Pleiades,
Or loose the band of Orion?
. . .
Knowest thou the ordinances of the heavens?
Canst thou establish the dominion thereof in the earth?
Canst thou lift up thy voice to the clouds,
That abundance of water may cover theee?
Canst thou send forth lightenings, that they may go,
And say unto thee, Here we are?[10]

[We have to be humble.]

I copied these words from *Voice Out of the Whirlwind,* and that is how I started my records.

* * * *

Upon entering The Room the next day, I found, lying in one corner and motionless, a young child. She seemed asleep, breathing lightly, her hands folded on her breast. I bent down to look at her face. She was pale with hollow cheeks; there was a death-like transparency about her. Her features were of pure design and great sensitivity. The blond hair was a tangle on her forehead. She was in rags and barefoot. Her feet were beautifully modelled and looked ani-

[10]Book of Job, 38:2 - 40:2.

mated like the feet of a dancer. I thought she was in her early teens, although her body was more a child's than a girl's. She looked neglected and half-starved.

I brushed her hair from her forehead, wondering who she might be and whether to wake her up. She turned her head under my touch and with a deep breath opened her eyes.

Her eyes were dark and of great depth. They looked hurt and scared. She did not smile. I talked to her gently, slipping my arm under her shoulders in an attempt to help her sit up. I asked her who she was and what she was doing here, had she gotten lost, and where were her parents? There was no answer. Her eyes seemed to go straight through me. The expression on her face was of a frozen stillness as if preserved under a transparent cover of ice. I didn't know if she saw or heard me.

I put my hand on hers and, with a soft caress, I asked her if she could get up. She sank back with her head against my shoulder, and her eyes closed again.

I looked around The Room, thinking that she needed food and a cover; her hands felt icy cold. I touched her bare feet, and they too were cold and bloodless. The Room was empty; there was no way of getting anything to eat. I thought I should try and lift her up. She would be more comfortable on the chair, and warmer. She would not be heavy, yet she was rather tall. I doubted that I could carry her. Maybe she was hurt and had to be picked up carefully. I was afraid to try it alone.

As I looked up from her, I suddenly saw the figure of a woman very close to me, behind a screen door, a dim shape, hardly recognizable in spite of her closeness. I gasped in terror. I had not seen the woman. It was uncanny. This sudden terror kept me motionless and speechless.

The woman pushed the door open and stood confronting me. I retreated to the far corner of The Room, with growing fear and an irrational desire to run. It was impossible to leave The Room. I could not see the door anymore. It seemed that my vision had grown dim. I tried to focus my eyes on the woman, but it was not possible to see more than her vague shape. She made a step toward the child, and I screamed.

But the woman gave no sign of recognition. I don't know if she knew I was there, clutching the curtain behind me and shaking. She bent down to the child, and then she looked up at me as with a silent request to come closer. I could not understand what frightened me so. I wanted to get out and go to U. Thinking of him gave me back some strength. I heard his voice within me. He said: Do not fear. I don't know how we got out and to the elevator. We must have carried the child between us. I cannot remember anything about it, but I found myself in U.'s room. The child was leaning against the door, looking at U.

I asked him where the woman was, but he had not seen the woman at all. Even when I explained to him that she had helped me carry the child, he shook his head—there had not been another woman. She will probably be back, he suggested, in her own good time. I told him how I had found the child sleeping, apparently half-starved, possibly hurt.

"She does not seem hurt," he said. He looked at her with great kindness, and under his regard life came to her face. I watched breathlessly. I had never seen anything more beautiful than the slowly opening blossom of this smile. It started in her eyes whose depth became luminous as an early morning sky under the kiss of the first ray of sunlight. It spread to her brow and over her cheeks in a faint blush, and at last her lips moved and parted. She did not speak, although the smile conveyed more than words could have told.

"She is lovely," I said. "How did you do it?"

"I don't know," he said. "I did not do anything."

"What are we to do with her? She should have some food."

"Yes, she might want milk."

U. took a glass and a pitcher full of milk from a cupboard and poured it for her. I was surprised to see him so well equipped for the emergency. He beckoned to her, but she made no move to come closer. "Take it to her," he said.

"I don't know. You better do it. She is so shy. She has smiled for you."

He went toward her with the milk, slowly, and with his eyes on her face. The gentleness of his gesture and expression gripped my heart: had anyone ever given to me in such a way? Who? When? He put the glass to her mouth, and it was like a caress. The child put her two slender hands over his holding the glass, and she drank avidly, looking at him in blank amazement.

"There," he said, "that's right. Won't you come and sit here?" He pushed a chair close to where I sat. The child did not move. "Maybe she does not understand English?"

"Assieds-toi," he said. Nothing. *"Setze Dich hin."* Nothing.

"Well," he said, "there she is. You better take care of her."

"I? How? What shall I do with her? Shouldn't we try and find her parents? She must belong somewhere, in a home."

"Maybe she is a foundling, maybe she has been left."

"Rather big for a foundling, isn't she? I wouldn't know what to do with her. I don't have time to care for a child these days. Don't you think I have outgrown that time in life? Why don't we try—there must be someone. Maybe call the police."

U. was picking up the telephone, but before he could dial the number, the child made a step toward him, hesitantly, then another, and then, with a great effort as if pushing herself forward against some resistance, with a swimming motion of her arms, she flew to his side and knelt by his chair, putting her head in his lap.

We were both so surprised that we did not say anything for a few minutes. Then U. slowly and thoughtfully lifted his hand and gently put it on her head.

"She is afraid," he said, "let's not call the police. You better take her along. We can find out later, when she has become less afraid. Maybe she will talk, maybe she knows where she belongs. You have room for her at your place, don't you? You told me you had rented a whole house."

"But I don't have time for children right now. I don't think I want her around. I need to be alone."

"Of course you have time. You don't want to leave her like that in the streets? It will be rewarding. She looks quite happy now. Isn't that nice? You take her home. We will see what to do with her later."

"I don't seem to have any choice," I said.

"No. You really don't have any choice."

It was difficult to make her leave. U. talked to her in a low and soothing voice, promising that she would be brought back the following day. I did not like the idea. To bring her back with me? I won't have any privacy with U. How could we work or even talk with her around?

"We will manage," he said.

He smiled at her and she slowly, hesitantly, got to her feet. At last we left. She did not mind walking in her bare feet. Her head was turned toward U. anxiously as I opened the door to let us out.

* * * *

The child had a way of disappearing which was difficult to figure out. It seemed that she had a keen sensitivity, though of another kind than what we are used to calling perception or intelligence. I thought she would be in my way and would need a great deal of care. But that was not so. She seemed to know when she was not wanted. I don't know what she did with herself at such times. She could not very well disappear into thin air, yet she ceased to be there and then appeared again in her own time. Maybe she was a nature-spirit, roaming through the redwood groves and nearby gardens, Ariel-like, on the wings of the summer breeze. Maybe she had hidden in a green corner, covered by the foliage of dense shrubbery, and gone to sleep. I could not know and soon gave up trying. She did not speak. There was no communication between us other than intuition. My thoughts about her seemed to touch her and move her, and she acted on them.

I set the table for her when I ate, and sometimes she took her seat across from me and nibbled at the food, and other times I called for her, and she did not come. She was very shy and savage. Her face was beautiful and blank, except for the times when she smiled. Her smile broke through like buds of cherry blossoms on the point of opening. But I did not know what would produce such a smile nor whether it was directed at me. I did not insist; I let her be, and at times I forgot her presence completely.

So all went well. She did not become a burden, and I did not have to leave my work on account of her. She was like a little wild cat, coming and going at her own whims. But she kept at a distance, though not in an unfriendly way. She withdrew when I wanted to touch her, and the hurt look came back into her eyes. So I desisted.

I put up a bed for her in the living room, and sometimes she would lie down and go to sleep while I sat by the crackling fire reading or writing my records. Other times she did not come to the living room at all, even when it got very late, but I found her there in the morning.

It was necessary to buy some clothes for her, and that presented a problem. She would not follow me into the store, but stood outside, looking at the things in the show-window. I got her several light summer dresses, pastel-colored and simple in make, and they set off her fragile beauty. They were just ordinary dresses as one would find for a youngster her age. But when I put them on her, they flowed down her graceful figure like a piece of breezy veil on a medieval angel. It occurred to me that she did look very much like a medieval angel in her unsubstantiality, and so I combed her light hair fittingly with the fashion of Chartres.

I had also bought a pair of soft slippers and some strong sandals for her beautiful feet, but she would not have them. Her feet behaved like little wild animals caught in a trap when I put the sandals on them. The toes wiggled, the arches rose as if in anger, and after a few seconds she got out of them with an impatient jerk. Yet her feet always looked clean, and in watching her walk I found her step so light that she seemed hardly to touch the ground.

"And what am I to make of all this?" I asked U. the next day. "You don't expect medieval angels to come to life and keep house with you? What kind of sense does this make? After all, we are living in the twentieth century. If anyone should see her around and ask about her, what am I to say? What about the Bureau of Records? She must have some civilian status. There ought to be some common-sense order about all this."

U. told me not to worry about these things. He did not know what to make of it either. It would all become apparent as time went on. There was no great probability that anyone would ask about her. Since she was so shy and withdrawn, she would keep away from strangers of her own accord. Maybe we could find out more once she could be persuaded to talk. She might tell us her story.

"I doubt that. It looks to me as if she does not have a story to tell. Maybe she spent her life sleeping, so she does not know what happened to her before. But I am not really so worried about people sticking their nose into this and asking about her. I am a stranger in the little town I live in, and I don't intend to make any acquaintances. What worries me is the uncanniness of the whole thing. To find her in The Room like this. How did she get in in the first place?"

"How does anybody or anything get into The Room?" he asked. "You must not forget that anybody appearing in The Room has always been there, somehow."

"What do you mean: somehow? That is just what I would like to know."

"Are you forgetting the nature of our Experiment?" U. asked patiently. "The Room is entrusted to you. It is your Room and your Experiment. It is your task to collect facts about The Room and work with whatever appears in it. These creatures, human, animal or plant, stone or element, are under your care. You must not regress to the intellectual mannerisms left over in our time. The Room has its own dynamics. Whatever is produced there has to be taken at face value. If you find a medieval angel, then you have to accept that figure into your life. As you have done. You have opened your life to include the figures in The Room, don't forget. It is not going to be your choice. You will not be able to make appear what you think you like or need. The laws are strict about that. What is there is there to exist. The Authorities are responsible, not you. You must have faith in the eventual outcome. I will help you. I will help you with everything that happens, however strange it may be. You can rely upon it."

Dear U., dear man, bless his heart. I have faith. It is really most exciting. I am fascinated. I shall be more patient and understanding. There is nothing I would rather do than work on The Experiment with him.

"She is nice," he said, "I like her. It should be possible to make her talk if we are patient."

The child was sitting on the floor in a corner of his room as we talked. She played with her toes and did not seem to pay attention to what we said. But at these words she looked up. I don't know how to describe what happened between U. and her. Neither of them moved. They just looked at each other. He smiled his good warm smile at her. Upon which she once more looked like a young fruit tree in bloom, dancing under a light summer breeze, leaves atremble. She got up as if under a spell and took a few steps toward him, and suddenly I saw that she was dance materialized.

"Yes," he said, as if in answer to my thought, "she dances beautifully. That too is language. We must try and understand that language."

At this, the child surrendered to some mysterious inner impulse and danced slowly, with ritual steps which seemed foreordained, going in circles upon circles toward U., approaching and retreating, until upon a gesture of his hand inviting her closer, she danced up to his chair and bowed down in deep reverence, her brow touching the floor, her hair falling about her, her arms open toward him. She remained in this position, swaying to an inner music inaudible to us.

It was of such beauty that tears came to my eyes. He too was deeply moved by the spectacle.

"She loves you," I said.

The child slowly raised her head. She looked at me and then at U.

"She loves you," the child said.

The miracle had happened: she spoke. It was not possible to know whether she had meant herself or me. Whether she said that she loved him, not knowing how to put it in the first person, or had she meant that I loved him?

She looked from U. to me and back at him.

"She has spoken," I said.

U. bent down to her and put his hand under her chin, lifting her face. "Yes, now she can speak," he said.

"Who are you? Where do you come from?" I asked.

But she did not seem to hear me. She was looking at U., and there was a deep surprise in her glance; she was overwhelmed.

"Yes?" said U. His voice was low, and the gentleness peculiar to him was in it. It was then that I realized for the first time this quality in U. He did not need to say much, and it did not matter what word he chose. There was in him a humanity of such depth and breadth that it would surely make a flower open under his very breath. His key word was simply: "Yes!" And it was yes to everything that is.

"She loves you," said the child, and her arms slowly closed as upon a new-found treasure she was taking to her heart. The emotion must have been too much for her. The flower drooped, and she sank to the floor, lifeless, as if in the sudden embrace of a deep sleep.

I felt my own love stirring within me, although I did not know how to hold it or acknowledge it. I was embarrassed, as I had been when the feeling first occurred after I had heard U. playing the *Appassionata,* the night of *Voice Out of the Whirlwind* speaking of humility and the human condition. I too felt tired. I thought I would now like to go to The Room. We agreed not to wake up the child, and U. assured me she could stay with him till I came back to fetch her.

* * * *

I must have fallen asleep in The Room as soon as I got down. I remember sitting down in the chair and closing my eyes. Immediately after that I was stretched out on a bed, and U. stood at the head of my bed. His presence made me happy with a happiness such as I had never felt. I reached for his hand, hesitantly, afraid that he might refuse to give it. But his hand came toward me, and then it came over my face like an embrace, covering my face and enveloping my whole being. There was in me a movement, opening me. As though a hand that had held me in its grip were loosening that grip. The circulation that had been stopped and dammed was allowed to flow. My inner organs, the inner bodily organs, were moving within me to the places where they rightly belonged. His hand was tenderly and carefully removing all obstacles and was moving aside the walls so that there was room, and into this openness I received his humanity.

A magic landscape opens. His hand is taking down the fences. All the fences are now being burned. There is a slow calm fire all over the fields. It keeps close to the ground, and it has a glow that illuminates the trees with their foliage, the birds in the trees, the flowers in their tenderness, the sky at the hour before dusk. The embers are even pebbles of black coal. And there are clean ashes which will go back into the brown earth for the coming year.

* * * *

I could not go to his room after this, and I forgot that I should fetch the child to take her with me. I somehow got into my car and drove home as in a dream, and I sat down to write into the records what had happened to me, as best I could.

"My blood sings with your speech. My heart grows with the look from your eyes. My soul spreads its wings on the breath of your spirit.

"What name do you have for such happening?

"I call it 'Love.'

"That is a good word. An old word. A new word. Love.

"But I am heavy with a dreadful fear. For I have written The Word.

"You know, U., my dear friend, I have never before been able to write the word: Love. Because that is the most dangerous and the most ridiculed and the most daring word.

"I feel about that word as the deeply believing Jews feel about the name of Jehova. You shall not say the Name. There is a sign for it, and they use the sign for the Name.

"I have never spoken the Word with my living voice. Twice in the course of my life have I whispered it, inaudibly, and so low that it was swallowed back into silence and the night, and it was not heard.

"But now I have written the Word, and it is addressed to U.

"As I wrote it, I feared that the letters would burn through the paper, and so it would not be there.

"But I remember that God came in a burning thornbush, and the bush flamed but was not consumed:

> And the angel of the Lord appeared unto him in a flame of fire out of the midst of a bush: and he looked, and, behold, the bush burned with fire, and the bush *was* not consumed. And Moses said, I will now turn aside, and see this great sight, why the bush is not burnt. And when the Lord saw that he turned aside to see, God called unto him out of the midst of the bush, and said, Moses, Moses. And he said, Here *am* I. And He said, Draw not nigh hither: put off thy shoes from off thy feet, for the place whereon thou standest *is* holy ground. . . . And Moses hid his face; for he was afraid to look upon God.[11]

"To love I say: Here am I. And I take off my shoes, because the place whereon I stand is holy ground."

* * * *

When I went to see U. the next day, I brought the records with me, but I was afraid to give them to him. I could not let him see the Word in writing, addressed to him.

I sat on my chair across from him, and I could not look at him nor speak. It was as if I had exchanged roles with the child. The sheets of writing dropped on the floor beside me, and I did not bend to pick them up, for I could not move. It was the child, whose presence in his room I had not even noticed till then, who picked up the papers. She took and collected the pages and gave them to U.

At this moment it became necessary for me to get up and withdraw to the far corner of the room, away from him, knowing that he would now see the Word in writing, naked and addressed to him. I thought, surely the Law will come down on me and crush me, for I have "drawn nigh hither."

But then I felt a light touch on my arm. The child was standing near me. She took my hand trustingly, and she led me back to my chair. When I could lift my head to look at U. I encountered his glance. He had read the Word. It was between us with the silent strength and beauty of the truth.

He said to me: "Yes. It is so. I shall take it and hold it in such a way that you can have it. You can trust me with it. I shall honor and value what is conveyed to me."

I could not speak. I returned his smile, and I fell into his eyes as into a deep well whence I could not return.

---

[11] Book of Exodus, 3:2-6.

Indeed, I was in the place of no return, and I was at his mercy. I realized a strong bond between myself and the child at this point. It seemed that only she could help me in this strange land. But she had not spoken again. Neither could I speak.

II.

At present, both my partner and I are in a fog. It is a light fog, so that we can hear and see each other. We can also understand what the difficulty is, but we have no way of handling it. As a consequence, it seems that The Experiment is interrupted. He says it is up to me to get it started again, but I am unable to do anything about it.

The disturbance is quite simply the fact that I cannot get a secure knowledge of my partner's reality. Can you imagine such a nonsensical thing? We sit there in his room where all the material is spread out, the test tubes are nicely stacked, the most recent solution is on the Bunsen burner, and I can hear its small hissing noise. He sits across from me in his usual relaxed way. We talk, yet I cannot know with security that he is there, that he is himself, that he is the same man who went with me through the time we call "before" and to which the records refer, that earlier time when the movement of the air he produced in putting his hand on his desk registered with me in a stirring deep down inside. It seems that this man is not the same. He is a stranger to whom I cannot get across anymore. Yet he is contained in the same body and has the same voice. All the evidence is in favor of his actually being the same man as the man I knew "before."

You see, visual evidence means so little. Knowledge means everything. My knowledge is transmitted to me through feeling, as I have said before. I can see he is the same. I can think he is the same, but I cannot know whether that is the truth or a trick, because I cannot feel it. As a matter of fact, when I ceased to feel his presence, I lost my sense of feeling altogether. So I am now without a compass and orientation.

Since I have lost the sense of feeling, I have also to some extent lost my voice. Not that I cannot speak at all. I can utter words and connect them logically. But an important element is missing. In the course of events "before," we had managed to produce a voice from within a clock. It had been a difficult part of The Experiment, maybe the most difficult part. There had been an old clock, one of those clocks in a wooden case that sometimes stand in people's living rooms, inherited from their great-grandparents. It is never wound up—its mechanism doesn't work anymore—and nobody tries to read the time it tells since its hands stay fixed and have always stayed at the same place as long as anybody can remember. Nobody would have thought about the clock at all except for the strange hint we got. We were told there was a voice imprisoned in that particular clock. I mentioned before it is always essential to follow up such messages. The message is usually contained in a hint given by The Authorities. The Authorities then expect us to do something about the thing hinted at. As a rule it is quite easy to take the first step. In this particular instance we had first to locate the clock. Well, it became apparent that I had the clock. It had stood in our dining room at home during the time of my childhood. That was a long time ago, and it is understandable that I forgot I had that antique. But, of course, you always have what you once had unless you take it and dispose of it. Otherwise it clutters up your attic or basement, and if too much stuff accumulates, it gradually overflows into the living quarters. I went searching for the clock, and there it was, stored away in a dark corner of the basement. I got it out, and we looked at it. My partner bent down a little to get a better view of the inside of the wooden case. Then, softly, he said, "Hello?" and the voice answered. It said, "Yes?"

So we knew there was this voice imprisoned in the clock. The next step was to liberate it. I could not have done that in a million years. But he did it. You see, that is only one of many things he was able to do in the period referred to as "before." I cannot tell you how he did it. It was with an inflection of his voice, with a hue of warmth, with a great concentration on liberating a thing that is imprisoned and should be alive. He did it with a very slight touch of his hand on the wood of the clock. He did it with the life-giving light in his eyes looking down into the case. The voice came out of the clock. A little voice. Very young. Very shy. A child of a voice. It was obviously a voice that had never been used, so it did not know how to make itself heard. It stayed silent, just hovering around us. He put out his hand, and as if the voice had just waited for this magic gesture, it alighted on his hand. He said something soothing. "There now, there you are." The voice started to vibrate. We could see its effort. It was quite moving to observe the young thing trying so hard to do something grown-up, making words. He was very sympathetic and understanding. Very patient. He knew exactly how it had to be treated. He also conveyed a feeling of great security. He said to this child that it should feel at home, that it was home now, that it was welcome. He instructed it in the art of making words come forth, saying that words are necessary as a Way toward understanding what it might need. You could see how neglected that child was. But it took in his encouragement avidly, and it saw the Way he was showing it, a Way that he made as he sat there, a wonderfully green path leading along a brooklet and with flowers growing along the borders. The child-voice at last let go of his hand and got onto the Way. And from there, among the flowers and close to the running water with its soft murmur, it spoke its first words.

What do you think were its first words? They were very low, almost a whisper, a breath between laughing and crying. It said, "I love you." And immediately, drunk with its new freedom, it said, *"Je t'aime—Ich liebe dich."*

We were both moved by the miracle that had happened, and we shook hands at this stage of The Experiment, with the silent understanding that we would take good care of this child. The Authorities were very pleased with us. We had worked it out to perfection. They said we would get an honorable mention for excellent performance. It was a bit difficult now since we were not alone any more. But little did we know how much more difficult it was going to get. The child needed so much care, and it had to be helped constantly. It became quite outspoken after a little while. The trouble was that its vocabulary remained very limited. All it could say was: I love you, *je t'aime, ich liebe dich.* He tried to teach it new words so that it could grow and develop, but it refused to learn anything else. It was contented with these words, and all it would agree to do was to add Italian and some other languages and say the same thing in all these languages. Well, we could not give it all this time and attention forever. We were busy carrying out the next messages and producing the next step. Somehow we must have forgotten about the child. I don't know at what point that happened. I might have to concentrate some time soon to find out where she got lost. At any rate, she did get lost. I was suddenly aware that she was missing. It was a great shock. It was understood that she was my responsibility. I had to look after her. I thought I had done the right thing by her. But obviously I hadn't. I noticed the lack when suddenly we needed her voice and it was not there. There was an important obstacle which could only be removed with the help of that little voice. He said, "I have done all I could in making her come out of that clock and teaching her to talk. If you let her get lost, you will now have to bring her back—she is your charge, not mine."

That is true. Yet, he too was fond of her. I pleaded with him to help me find her again. But he flatly refused. We got into an argument about it. We are still held up by that argument. And since the voice disappeared, the most important words are missing. The argument can't be settled. At this point the fog started to roll in, and the whole thing resulted in the complete loss of identity I referred to when I explained that I lost my bearings.

* * * *

Something important is happening this very minute, and I have to interrupt to tell you about it. I found the child. Just as I spoke about losing my voice and having an argument with my partner, an argument in which I could not support my own side well enough since the necessary words were missing, I found the child.

I found her in a dark corner of this very Sunday. I came back from a short walk to buy a can of soup for supper. I had been writing all day, and as I looked up from my paper, I was suddenly aware of the bright sunlight, the clear day, the fresh breeze. I noticed how quiet my room was and that I had not spoken to a living person for a very long time. So I went outside to go to the store. The streets were empty. Cars drove by, and there were people in them who were spending this Sunday together, and they looked contented. I walked slowly, taking in the air and the people and my own keen sense of loneliness. I thought of age approaching, and I thought of having to face the long days and nights alone. I thought of him, my partner, spending the day with his family. I wished him well. I hoped it was a good Sunday for him.

I thought how "before," at the time of those early records, I had spent many a Sunday with him. He had allowed me to summon his presence. It was during the time I used to call my first marriage to him, and after the child had been produced. She was with us then. Her desire and her love were so strong that I was not even aware of his not being present in actuality. We talked to him. We heard his voice answering. We sat at his knees, and we caressed his hair and his temples. Oh, we were happy.

I am too horribly lonesome since the child disappeared. And

maybe this is the first time since she got lost that I have thought of her with emotion. So this is how I found her: at this Sunday's darkest corner, lying quietly, her hands folded over her heart. I thought she was sleeping and bent closer to put a cover over her and smooth her hair which was all a tangle on her forehead. I noticed that her face was cold, and I bent still closer to listen to her heartbeat. A terrible fear gripped me. But she opened her eyes and smiled at me, a smile that cut to the core. Her little body felt very slight. "Are you hungry?" I asked her. She nodded, but as I wanted to get up to warm the soup for her, she caught my arm with a thin transparent hand.

"No," she said, "don't go away. If you go away you might forget me again."

"Never," I said. "I shall never forget you again."

"It is too late," she said, "I have to go. There are only a few moments left."

"No," I cried, "never. You must not go. I cannot be without you. You will be well again. I will take care of you. Oh, but you must believe me, please. I haven't really forgotten you. I just could not remember clearly enough. I could not see you. There was so much fog. I lost you in the fog. It will never happen again—we will never part anymore."

She smiled. "Thank you," she said, "that makes it easier. I must go now. But I will leave my voice. You may use it to speak of love. Don't forget."

"But he does not want to hear of love. We have spoken of love too long. He wants to hear of other things."

"That is not true. He will want to hear whatever it is we say. Don't forget. If you don't speak of love anymore, nothing will be left of me. I do not want to die in eternity. I leave the voice in your care. To speak of love."

These were her last words. There was no fight; death came like a caress over her face. Her smile was the smile of L'Inconnue de la Seine. Her face had become that girl's eternal face, in sweetness.

And so I must accompany her to her place of rest. We do not have to go far. I know the place. It was a place she liked to visit: Margaret's.

Nor mouth had, no nor mind, expressed
What heart heard of, ghost guessed:
It is the blight man was born for,
It is Margaret you mourn for.

Mourning, I shall talk to him of Margaret.

Margaret, are you grieving
Over Goldengrove unleaving?[12]

My words will be clad in her voice, and there never need be any argument. He will want to remember her, and she will be safe with her light death between the stanzas of the poem.

And now, she has had her short span. Now, do I have to go back to the black sea of loneliness? I do not know the answer. The central problem remains: how to find the mysterious U.?

"In the meantime I may be of help perhaps," said a voice.

I looked around the room. Leaning against the window, a book in his long slender hands, stood the Painter.

"It has been a long time," I said. "Welcome in America. I am happy to see you safe. How did you find me?"

"I have to give that question back. How did *you* find *me?* I was told to come. So here I am."

"It is true, I have been thinking of you lately. But there was so little hope of finding you. I was afraid you might be dead—that they caught up with you."

"You are too easily afraid."

"That may well be. Your hands, you have kept your hands!"

"Yes. It is my eyes."

"Your eyes? What happened to them?"

"I am blind."

"Oh—"

"It does not matter. I could paint without them."

"How is that possible?"

"With your help."

"I do not understand."

He laughed and came toward me, his step was light and firm. He took my arm and asked me to lead him to a chair. "I will know this room in a short while. It will be easy."

I made him comfortable, and leaning back he explained to me that I was to write out his painting. It will be a sketchbook.

"But I am busy right now. I am writing an important report. I cannot find time for anything else."

"I know about the records you are keeping. The Authorities have

[12] Gerard Manley Hopkins, "Spring and Fall: To a Young Child."

assigned me to help you. There might be a connection between the sketchbook and these records."

I was silent for a long while. This was very confusing. How could a third person be allowed to know, and how could he understand?

"I really don't know. I cannot imagine how it can be done. I am not that kind of writer. I just want to report facts."

"We will see. You must not fear that I will intrude. You don't have to explain anything. You can use me for the stage settings. You will find that you can use me for most anything, chiefly to keep you company. I have been told you are lonely. I too am lonely."

"I am glad you came. You know that, don't you? There will be time for the sketchbook, I am sure. But it must be postponed."

He agreed to wait, and shortly afterward he left.

When I told my partner about it, it seemed so strange that I was not quite sure anymore whether it had happened at all. He could not explain it, but he was quite pleased about it.

"The child leaves and the painter comes in," he said. "It is not so strange, really. It makes sense."

So I saw that he already knew about the child's death.

"I am sorry," he said, reading my thought. "I am sorry it had to happen this way. But I know that she has left her voice. I will be glad to hear her voice, you need not fear." I thanked him. We were silent. There was nothing to say. He asked me if I were still mourning her.

"I had not known it was Margaret," I said.

"Margaret—and L'Inconnue de la Seine," he said, " 'Spring and Fall: To a Young Child.' There will be new tasks. The next step."

But I am not ready for the next step, I am afraid. He explained to me that I had already taken it. I had made the step when I buried the child.

"I love you," I said. But it was not the child's voice, nor was it Sulamith's; neither was it my own voice. It was a new and unaccustomed voice.

"You see. You can speak again. That is good."

"Where do we go now?" I asked.

"I don't know," he said.

"What do we do now?"

"I don't know," he said. "We must wait. It will become clear." It is terrible to wait. My patience is worn thin. Time is heavy on my hands. Am I still in the desert?

III.

U. had died. I was told about it in a dream. The dream was saying it carefully, in a hidden way at first, just hinting that somebody had died. I asked who had died but could not get a straight answer. It was as if they wished to prepare me slowly, for it might easily kill me. And then, in a manner which I cannot describe, it became clear that it was U. who had died.

I screamed in the dream, and it must have been a blood-curdling scream, for the night nurse came running. When she woke me I was in tears, although I did not remember why I was crying. She gave me a sedative which did not put me to sleep, nor did it stop the crying. But it must have relieved the impact of the message when it dawned on me.

This same night I died myself. Nobody was there at my bedside, and the agony of the interminable hours was impenetrably black and solid with the solidity of immovable rock piled over my heart. There was no consolation and no comfort. There was no movement within or outside. It was the petrified silence and immobility of death, and even my tears had stopped flowing.

I don't know how many days and nights it lasted; there did not seem any awareness left of things external. They must have gone on treating me as though I were still living, taking care of what needed to be done around a sick person's bed. But I have no memory of it, nor of whether I spoke or ate or moved.

I knew I was in my grave and dying, and I knew I should have been dead before being buried. I thought it could not last eternally, that the relief of complete extinction would come soon, but I cried to God and repeated the same words which have come to us across the ages to express the utmost despair of the soul and the body:

My God, my God, why hast thou forsaken me?

No answer came.

The pain of his death was so great that it numbed me, and I could not think of him. I could not go near that thought. At that thought the world had come to an end, and life had ceased, and my blood had left me. There was the emptiness of the void where the solid and the liquid had not been separated, and the breath of God had not created light to pierce the darkness. After the end it was as it had been before the beginning. And the spirit of God did not hover over the waters.

Oh, but do you know the place where God ceases? It is the eternal abyss of night whose air is moved by the fruitless howling of wolfish winds and where there is no growth but that of ungiving stone whose vegetation does not have the juice of life nor does it bleed in the pain of death. Can you think of rocks weeping? You cannot.

And therefore in this place even the bitterness of tears seems sweet with the grace of living. But tears are swept off your face in this place, and only their knife-sharp traces are left to bite your skin.

And in this place of non-being which is not yet the place of Death himself, there is towering over the abyss God's inhuman shadow, the great Absconditus.

Oh my beloved, and I could not see his face, nor even remember. Memory was extinguished, and I did not know his form nor even his name, and I could not call to him, for it was as if I had never known him. I could not mourn his death, for he had never lived.

I don't know what manner of pain I felt other than the unbearable anguish of a slow petrifaction. Yes, I turned into stone, and I was aware of this transformation from my toes up through my body, slowly moving closer to my heart. And as I felt the stony hand creeping over my flesh, I knew that it would reach my heart soon and that the unbearable anguish was not yet really unbearable, for there would be the moment of feeling my heart turn to stone and the last breath yet moving through my lungs and the next second of the ceasing heartbeat and the breath arrested, stifled in stony stillness. And I lay there and feared that moment with a fear so great that I could not contain it, and with a hopeless desire that the last second may be granted before the last second, immediately.

And suddenly the fear let go of me, and I submitted to my death. My memory came back, and I knew that I had lost him, that he had once been there but was not there anymore.

I thought it would be a great blessing to be dead, even if I first had to die to then be dead. Rather than live through the eternal damnation of stone, knowing that he had died and that I was left. Nobody needs to do what he cannot do, and when you come to the place where all is stopped, you are graciously allowed to cease. It was this thought that gave me comfort. I submitted to my death, and I could patiently wait for it to complete itself. God had after all not forsaken me. He relieved the unbearable and made it cease. Something rather close to peace came over me at this recognition that I was being dealt with in fairness.

It was at this point that U. came.

There was a knock at the door which I knew I could not and need not answer, for I was unable to make myself audible, and I did not open my eyes to see who was coming. In the grave one has achieved this sublime indifference. But then I heard his voice.

How can I describe to you the eternity of that moment of pain in trying to recall one's soul from the state of non-being, to open one's eyes and send forth a glance which has to travel through limitless space to arrive at the specific setting in which was placed my deathbed? It took the utmost force of persuasion to believe I had heard his voice, and then it took the utmost strength to lift the heaviness of my lids so that the far-travelled glance may cross the border to the land of the living. I saw him standing at the head of my bed.

I saw that he was there and was living. It was his face with his deep kind eyes. It was his wide generous mouth saying to me I don't know what words, but moving his lips, his hands lightly taking mine and passing on. It was he, and he was living. I knew then that I too would live.

Did I speak with him? I cannot remember. There are events of the soul which cannot reach words, and the miserable limitations of human strength do not permit one to embrace a moment like that in fullness. I saw that he was living, and I saw that he stood by my bed, and his death had been but my own death in passing to another form of life. It had been the death of my requests made to life which could not be fulfilled and which had to die.

I did not have these thoughts so clearly at that time. I only knew that he was there, sharing with me the air of the room I lay in, and visible in the light of day coming through the window as through an opening in my grave. I could not lift myself out of the confining embrace of that grave, but I could see him and perceive the light in which his form stood out, and I could draw in the shared air, and that was all, and that was enough, and it was rebirth, and it was resurrection.

Since that moment, and for the weeks and months of my convalescence, I had the knowledge that it was enough that he was living. Is it that one has to be deprived so completely before the deepest knowledge of the essential can become clear?

In this way I have learned obedience. Not of my own free will and not by choice. Not at all because of some great inner strength and humility. Not at all. Obedience was forced upon me with the threat of death and the actual experience of death. And it is death which awakens in the soul an undiscriminating gratitude to life. And do you not believe that this may be the meaning of death, to become aware of life in the deepest sense?

I do not say that I am now able to forego the requests of my body and soul to be given happiness and fulfillment. The obedience I spoke of is not a thing one may acquire and keep without struggle. This obedience to life and to the reality of fact in one's life is but a ray of light by which to orient my steps, and it still grows dim at times, and it is threatened by extinction at times. It is an endless task to be learned anew every day. But I hope it will become easier as time goes on, and that there will be developed a faculty for it with which to recall it, to relieve the passion of my soul for U.

It would be false to say that I understand and have found justification for the facts of my life, which are that I be without fulfillment. I do not. I do not understand, and I cannot justify. And I cannot forgive God for making it thus and asking this.

But I have learned that neither life nor God—and they are one and the same to me—care whether we understand or justify. There is a great severity and hardness in life and in God, and our questions and our rebellions are not indulged. Maybe it is that our life is not made to please or displease. Maybe there is a law by which it can be understood, so that you can perceive a goal it is leading to and a meaning to be accomplished. It is infinitely comforting to believe that, and I shall believe it. That would make it possible to set forth on the exploration of the ultimate goal and meaning. This is what I wish to do now. And again I must say, for the sake of truth, I have not come to this decision by my own free will; it has been forced upon me. I trust that U. will be with me in this pursuit, which is not the pursuit of happiness.

It is sweet and kind of the men who formulated the Immortal Rights to say that one of them is the pursuit of happiness. But I believe that right cannot be granted to man by man. It might be a mistake to believe that life makes any such promise. It is surely a wrong premise. The pursuit of happiness is an inborn need and faculty. But that is all. No promises are given, and no promises are therefore broken.

It must have been this error which led me through death toward a new clarity. I insisted that there be fulfillment for me, and I felt justified, not having done anything to deserve what I thought to be the punishment of denial. And with this good conscience, I set out to make for myself the fulfillment that was needed, and to which I thought I had a right. To give this up seemed like giving up life. And, in making it where it was not, I almost killed U. and myself within my soul. There was this terrible strength within me to make real and concrete that which was not real and concrete and to bring about the miracle.

But this is Easter time, the time of the Opening of the Grave and the Resurrection of the Living Essence. We may not perform miracles, but miracles may be performed in us. And U. has come back to me, and his hands briefly took mine, and his smile lighted up the desert of my soul, and life started moving, and through the stone broke the green stem and the red flower of love renewed.

My heart has grown one pain deeper and one knowledge wider. That I have seen the miracle of stone putting out a blossom. That I have felt the non-life of that which is stone. That water can spring from rock if God touches it with his wand. And that I have lived through the life and damnation of our brother stone. I am not asking anymore whence this love came, nor why I have it, nor why it chose to settle in my heart. It is there, and it has survived one big and hard and incomprehensible death, after surviving many smaller life-size deaths. Who am I to ask such questions and demand such answers?

I shall live with this love and not request that it bring me happiness, nor that it bring me anything. If I am found worthy to be its abode, I shall keep home for it as if it were he I am keeping home for. I pray that God keep him and protect him, and that he may not step out of sight.

It is better to live with love than to live without love.